Though he be but little, he is fierce

~ William Shakespeare
paraphrase *A Midsummer Night's Dream*

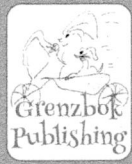

BRAVE LIKE LUKAS
THE LITTLE PUP WHO FACED HIS FEARS

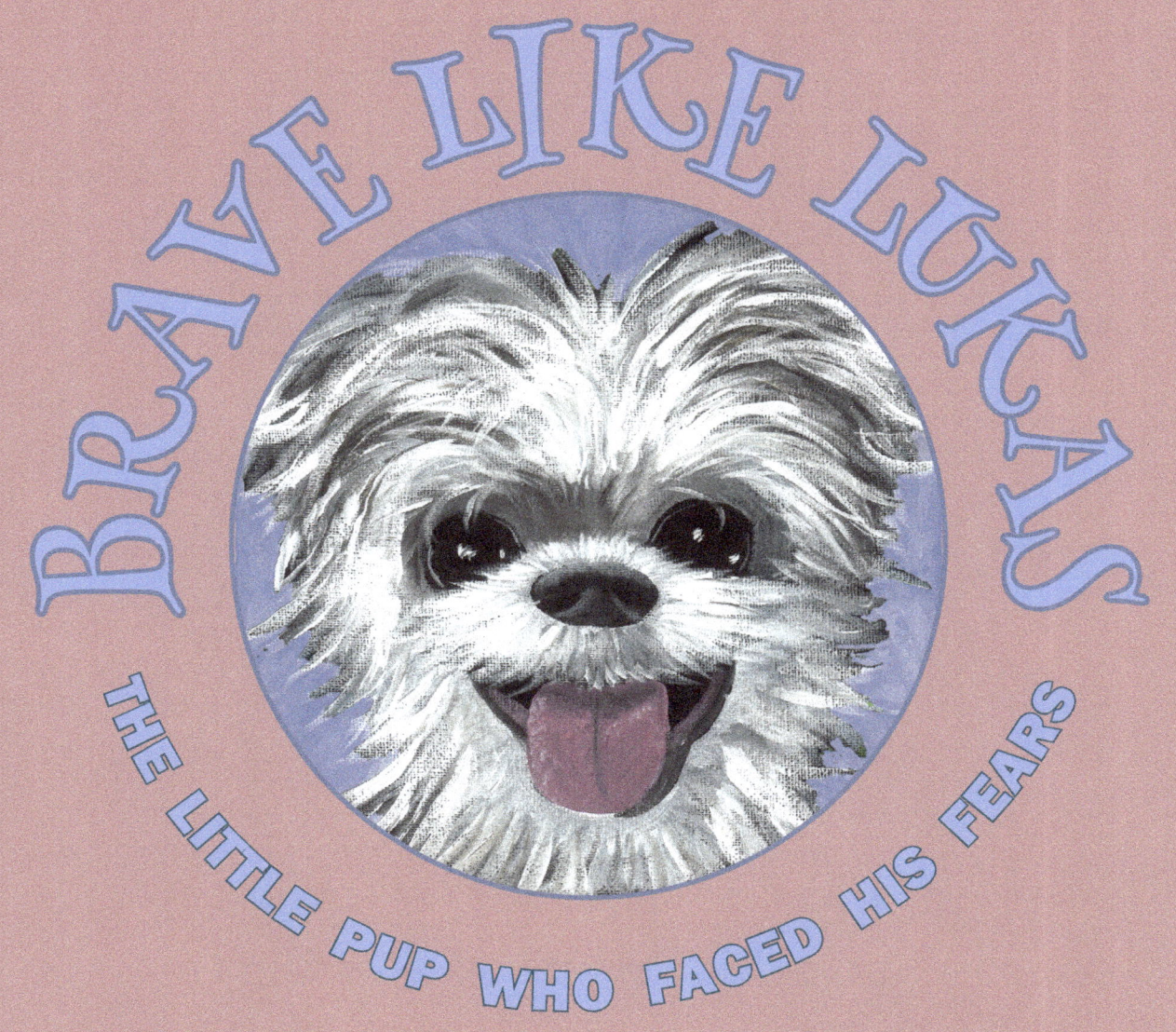

LISA MARIE RUSSELL
ILLUSTRATED BY CLAUDIA KRISSINGER

Copyright © 2025 Lisa Marie Russell

ISBN 979-8-9926589-2-7
Printed in the United States of America

All rights reserved. This book or any portion thereof may not be reproduced or used in any manner whatsoever without the express written permission of the author except for the use of brief quotations in a book review. For permissions, contact Grenzbok Publishing.
The story herein is not intended as medical or veterinary advice. This is just the tale of one very brave little dog.

Grenzbok Publishing.
www.grenzbokemail.comcast

CREDITS

Paw prints, https://www.freepik.com/free-photos-vectors/dog-paw-print">Image by starline</a> on Freepik

Portrait of author and pets, Debora Cartwright, Del Mar Photographics.
All other photos property of author

Illustrations: Claudia Krissinger: claudiakrissinger.wixsite.com/petportraits

Book and cover design by Maureen Moore, Booksmyth, Shelburne Falls, MA

Dedicated especially to
Nanny/Mom who was
brave like Lukas

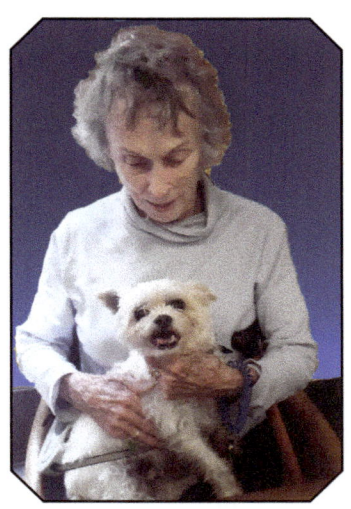

and to Dad, Pete,
and Max,
my first pack

We are grateful to all our many friends
who have been so encouraging —

Dale Baker, Jay Barrett, Mare Biddle, Robin Brande, Audrey Campbell, Marilyn Dupree, Jane Diers, Judy DiMeo, Brian Fix, Jess and Lucille Goodman, Laurie Gunn, Claudia Krissinger, Bonnie Lorden, Lynn McCoy, John Miskec, Maureen Moore, Maria Munroe, Laureen Ryan, Sharon Thomerson, and Sue Wallace.

Special thanks to

Dr. Kirk Feinberg, who took such good care
of us and never gave up;
Vet Tech Lena Griffith, who was so kind
in showing us what to do;
Sue, Anita, LeAnn and all Lukas' girlfriends at
Governor Animal Clinic who show him so much love;
and Chihuahua Rescue of San Diego.

WOOF!!!
Hi! My name is Lukas!

What's your name??

I'm a little white and tan pup with big brown eyes and ears that flop over sometimes. I'm a Chihuahua-mix little doggy. I only weigh nine pounds!!!

I smile a lot. Mom says I'm very cute!!!

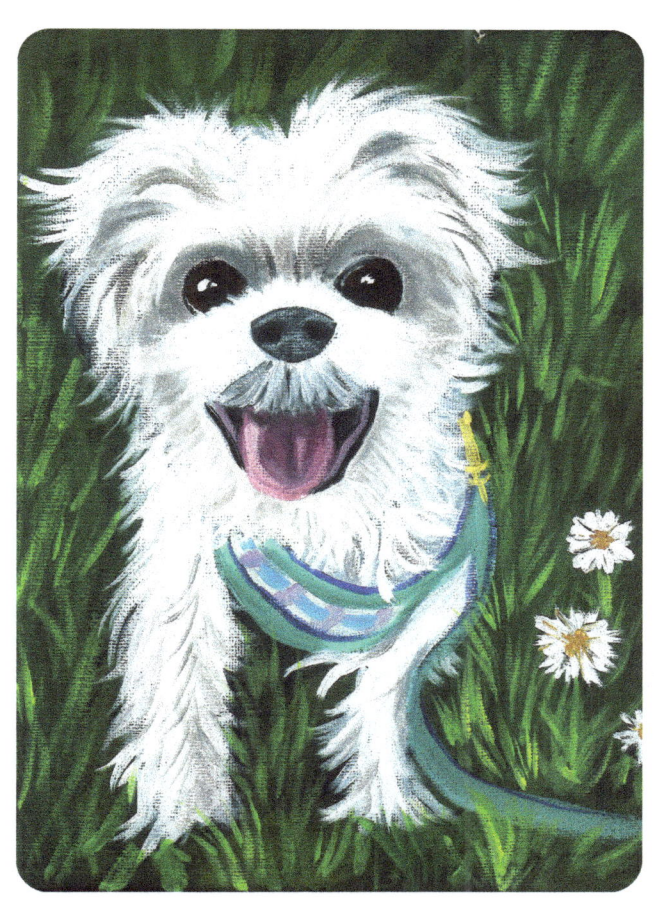

I have lots of different looks! Sometimes I have long hair and then after a haircut, I have short hair. And sometimes I'm in between!

Sometimes one of my ears is up, sometimes both are up, and sometimes they are both floppy!

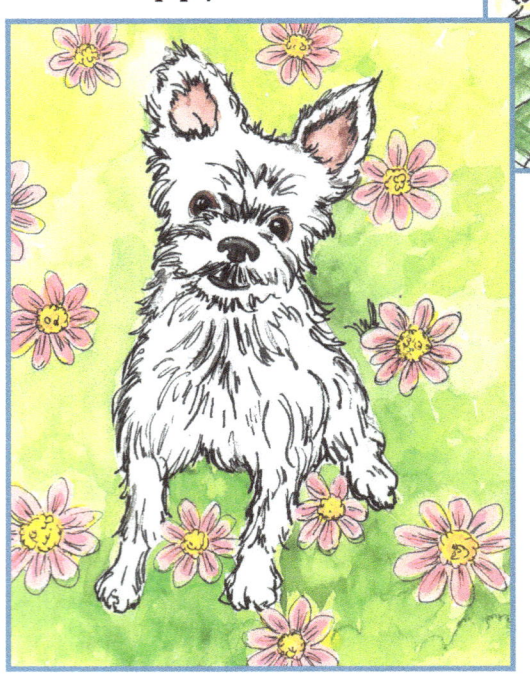
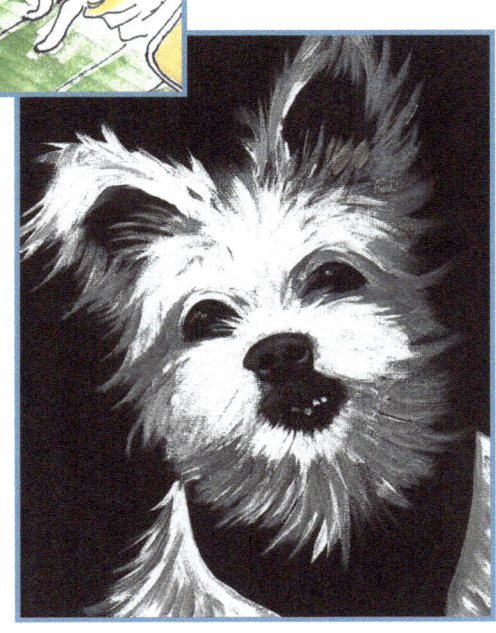

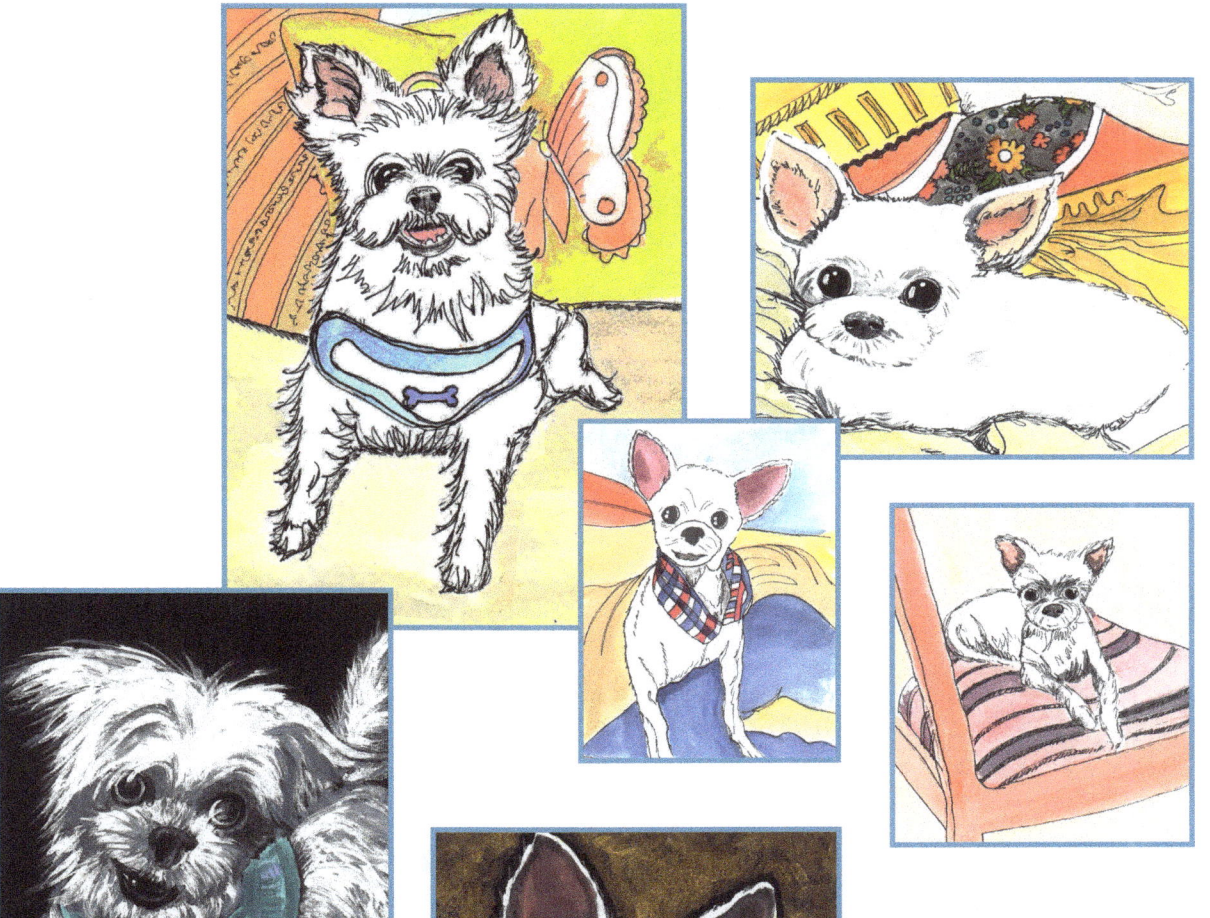

Which one is your favorite look?

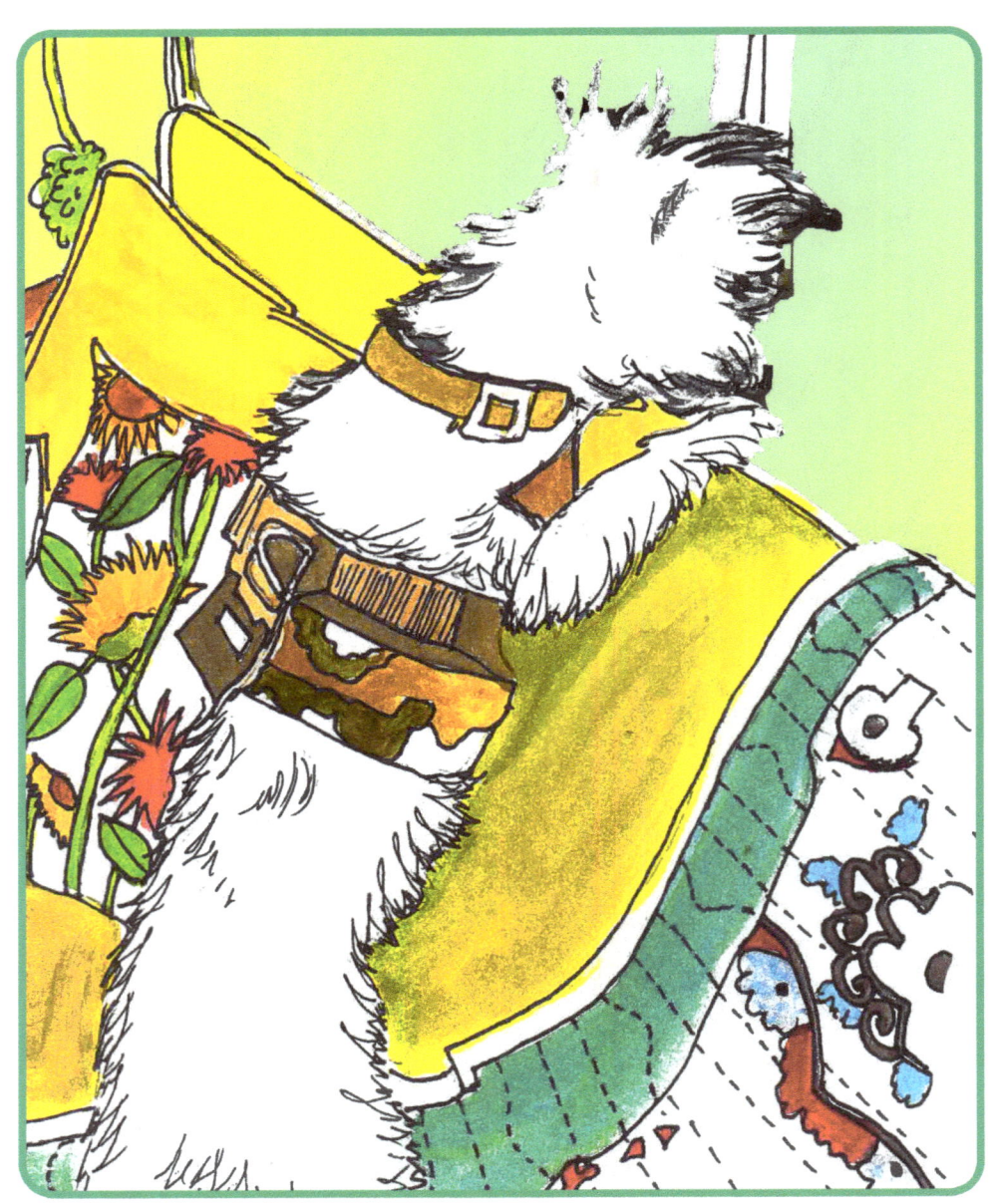
GUARDING THE HOUSE

Mom says I am a very loyal and thoughtful little dog. I guard the house and follow her around to make sure she is all right.

I always greet her at the top of the stairs when she comes home.

I take my jobs very seriously!!

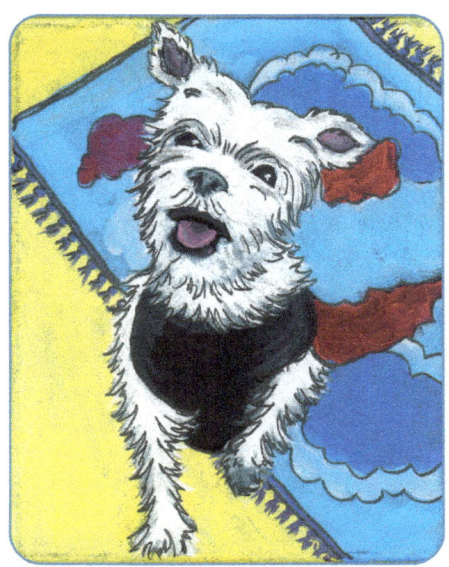

KEEPING AN EYE ON MOM

Mom has all kinds of silly nicknames for me, like **Bubs**,
     Papa Smoosh,
          Jelly Bean Nose,
               and even **Lukie Patookie**.

Do *you* have any silly nicknames?

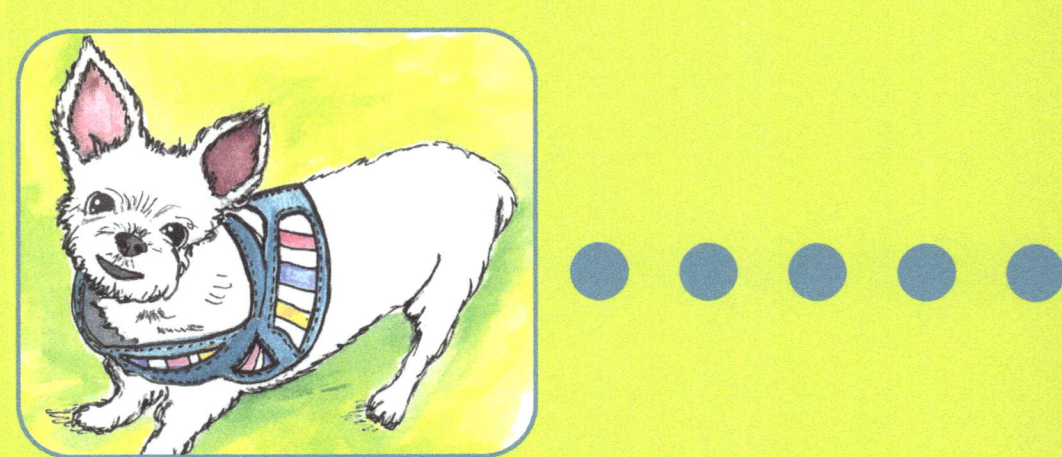

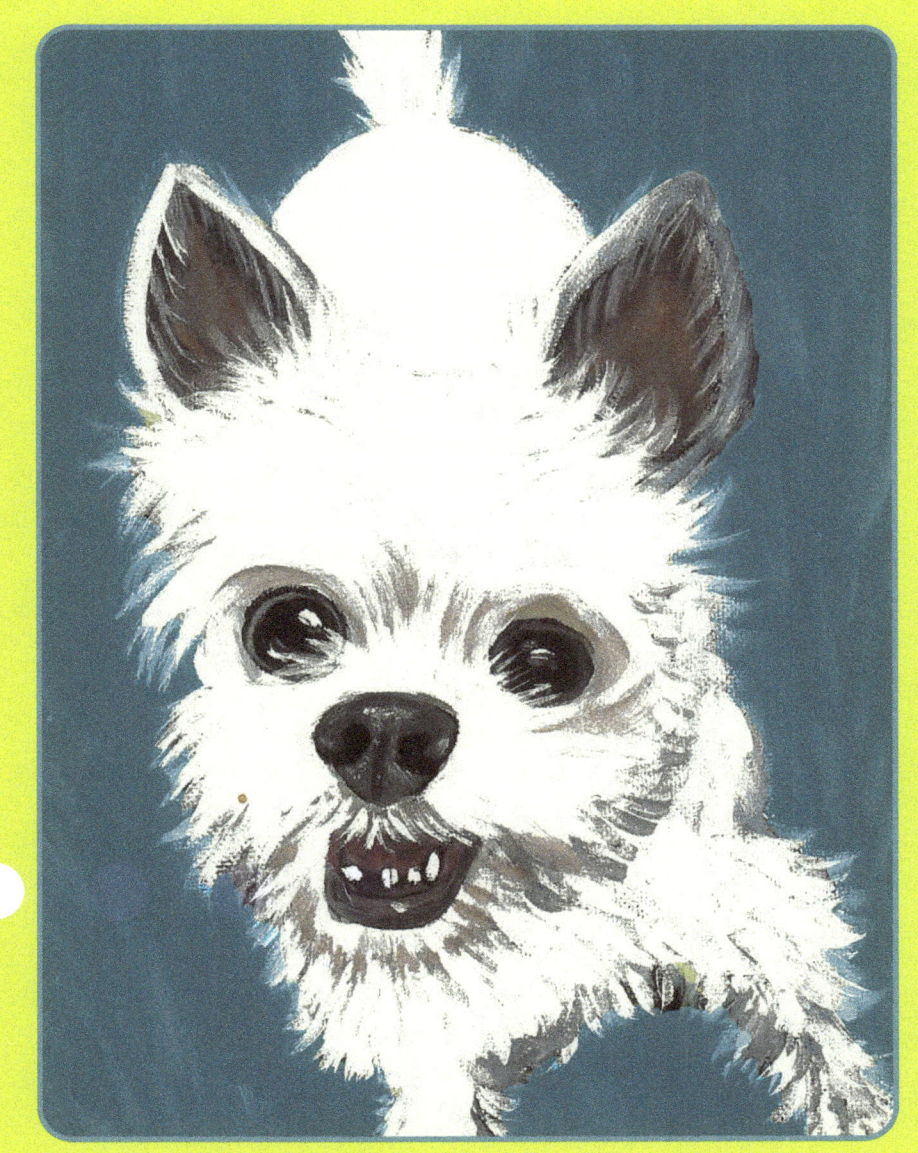

I live with my mom, two other dogs named Tica and Kai, and six kitties named Penelope, Tippy, Murray, Jasper, Tweed P. Fluffington, and Zeke!

We all live in a very colorful and cozy house.

Do you and your friends have any pets?
What kind are they?
What are their names?

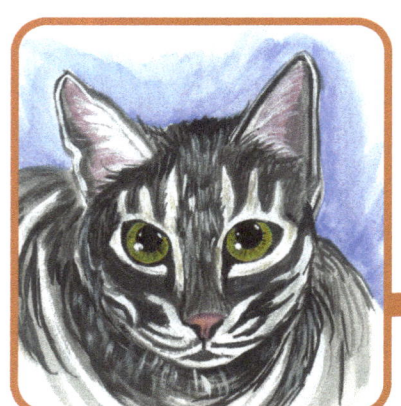

TWEED P. FLUFFINGTON

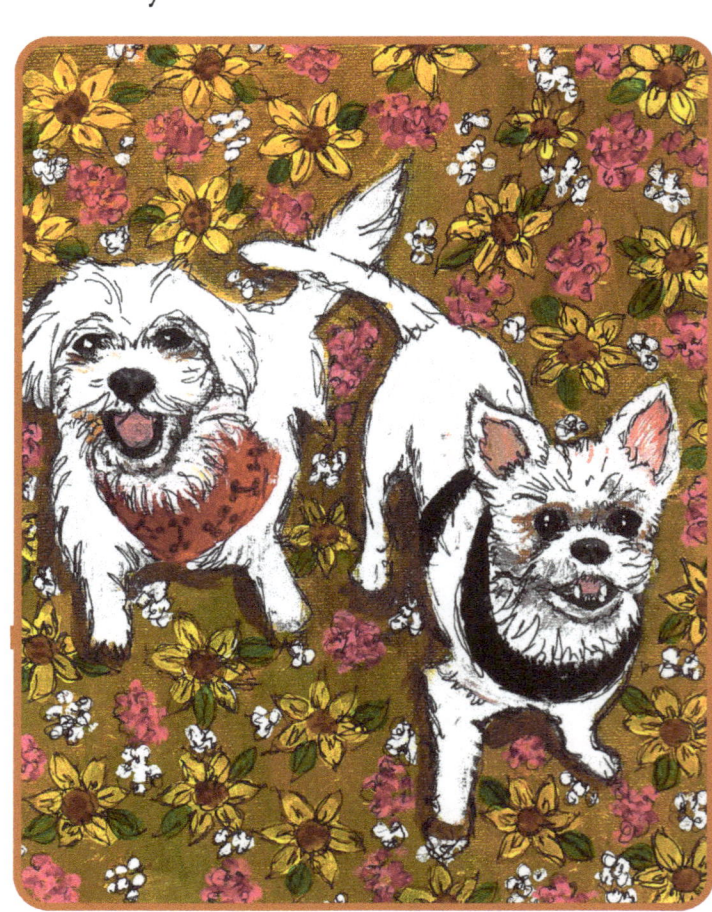

KAI AND ME

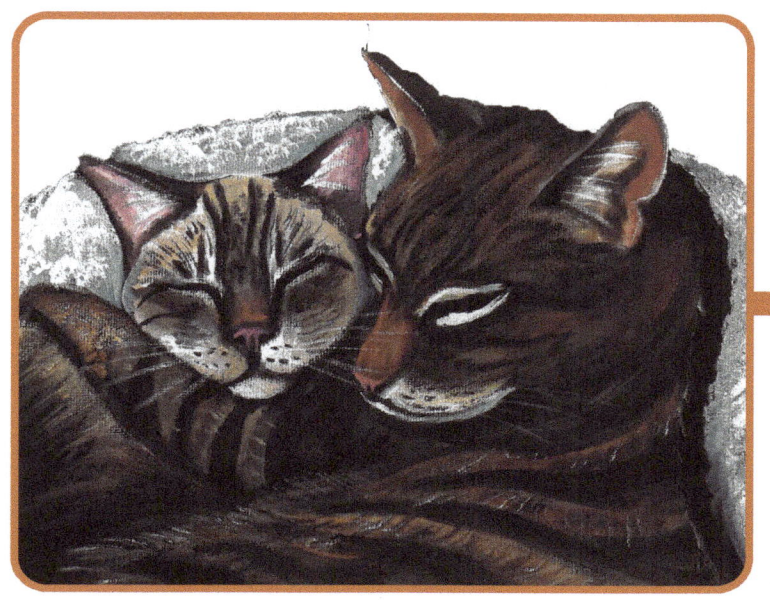

MURRAY AND JASPER

TICA AND ZEKE

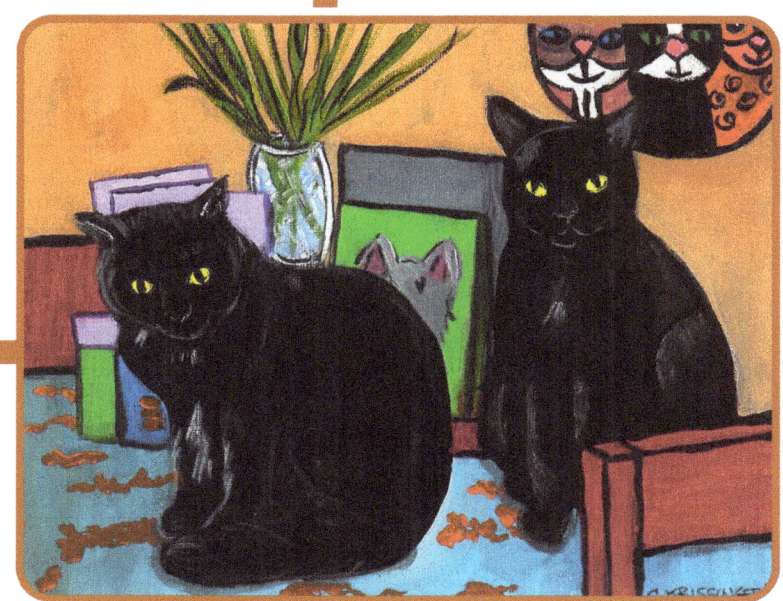

PENELOPE AND TIPPY

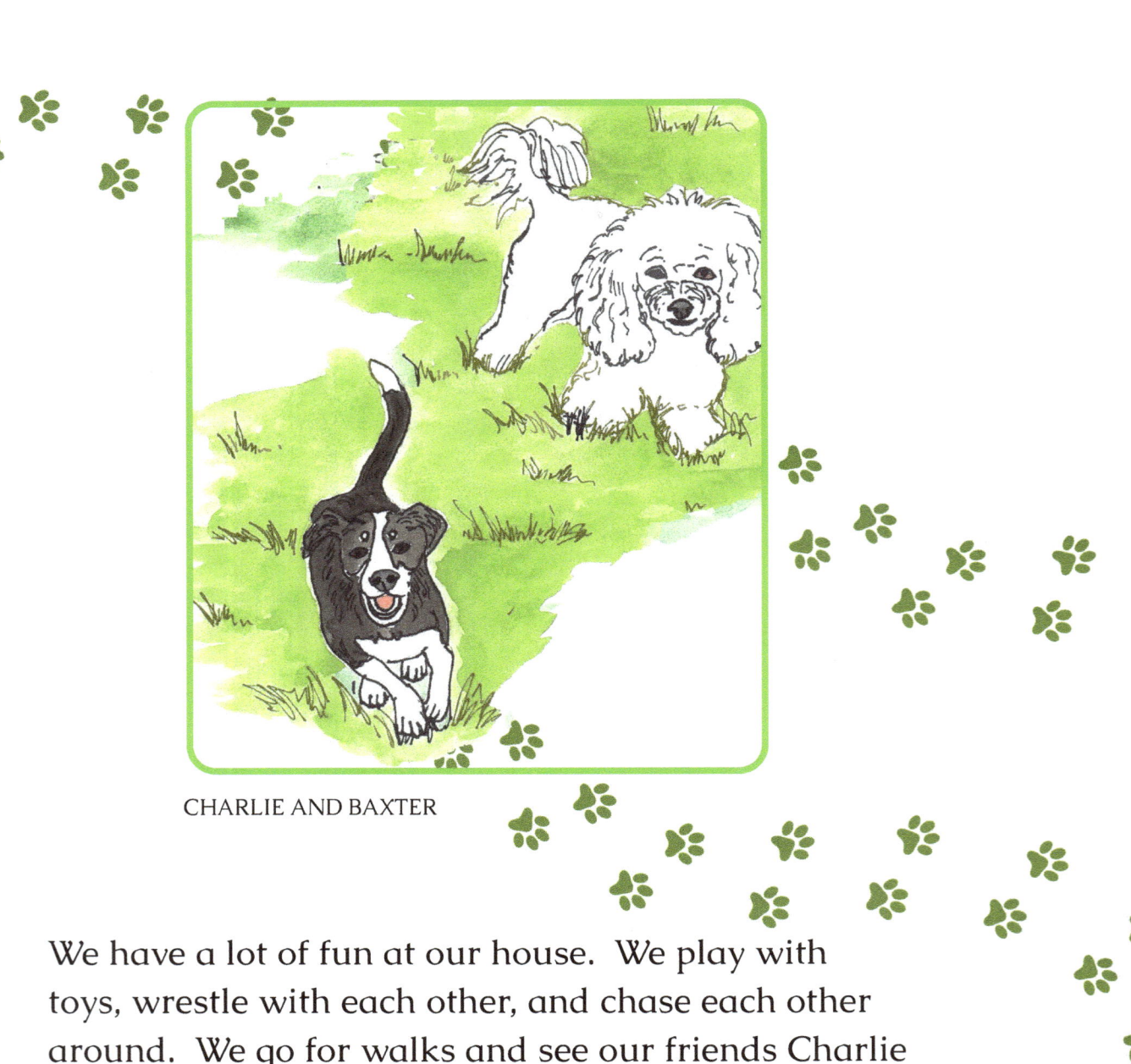

CHARLIE AND BAXTER

We have a lot of fun at our house. We play with toys, wrestle with each other, and chase each other around. We go for walks and see our friends Charlie and Baxter along the way.

Our kitty, Murray, comes with us on our walks! He rides in the stroller with Tica while Kai and I walk.

Have you ever seen a kitty go for a walk with some pups??

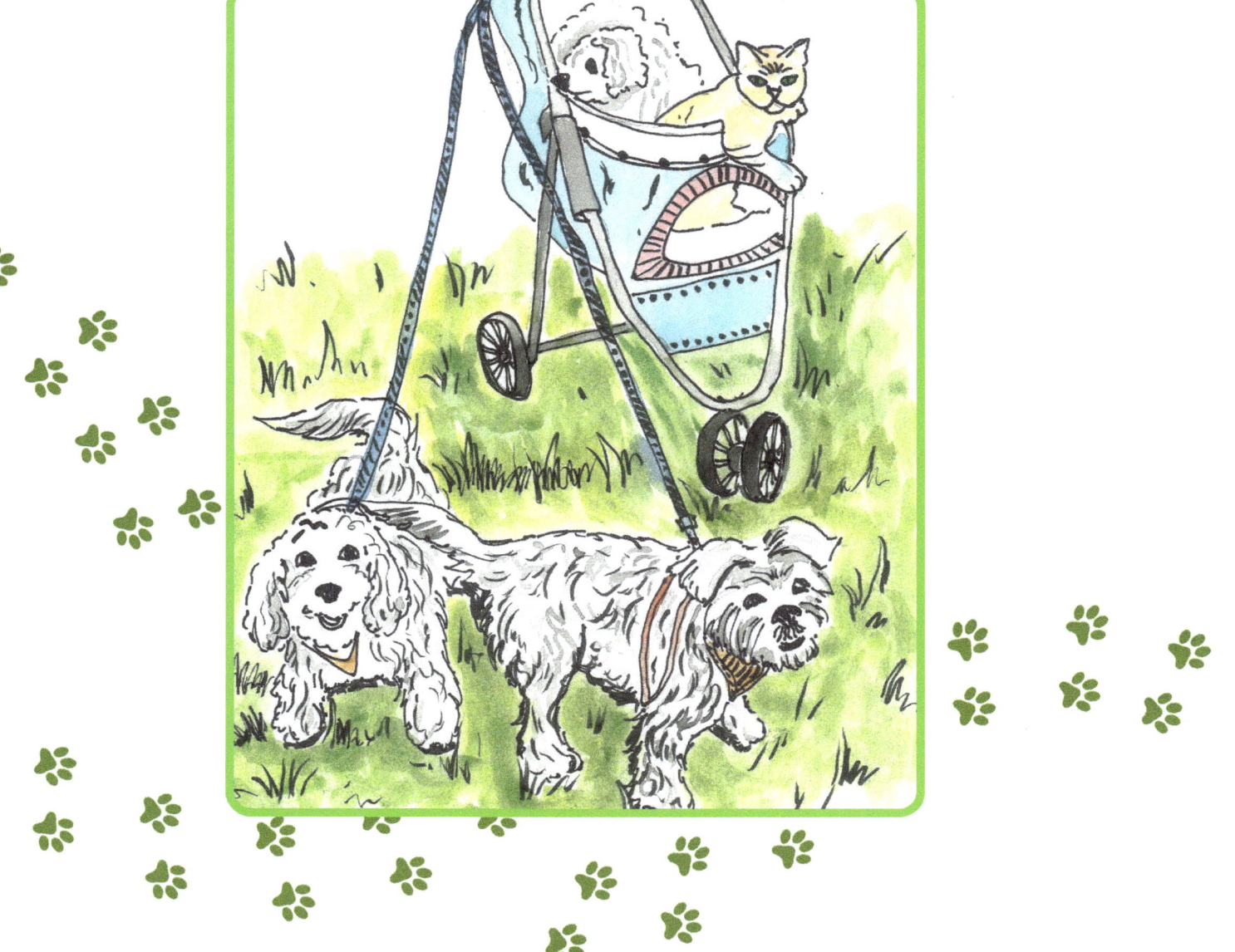

My mom says she loves us to the moon and back. She works really hard to make sure we are happy and healthy. We eat good food and go on long walks every day to stay in shape.

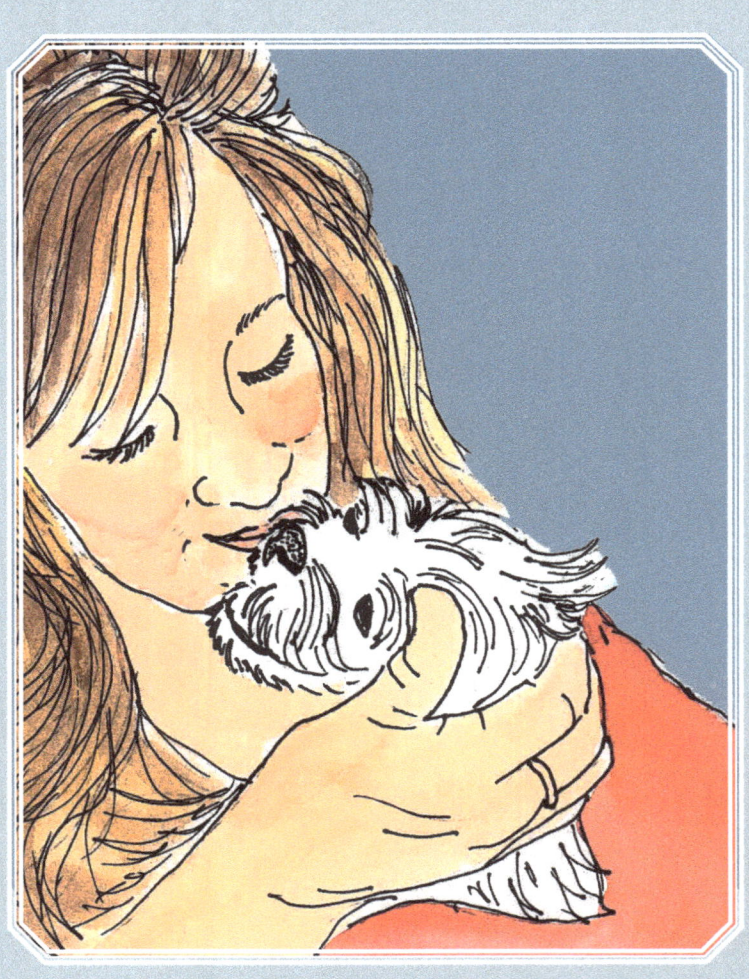

But even with all that, one day I did not feel well. My stomach hurt and I had no energy. I was very thirsty and felt grouchy and confused. I did not want to play with my toys or wrestle with my sisters or chase the kitties. I didn't even want a treat!!! Mom was scared.

Have you ever felt sick? What did it feel like?

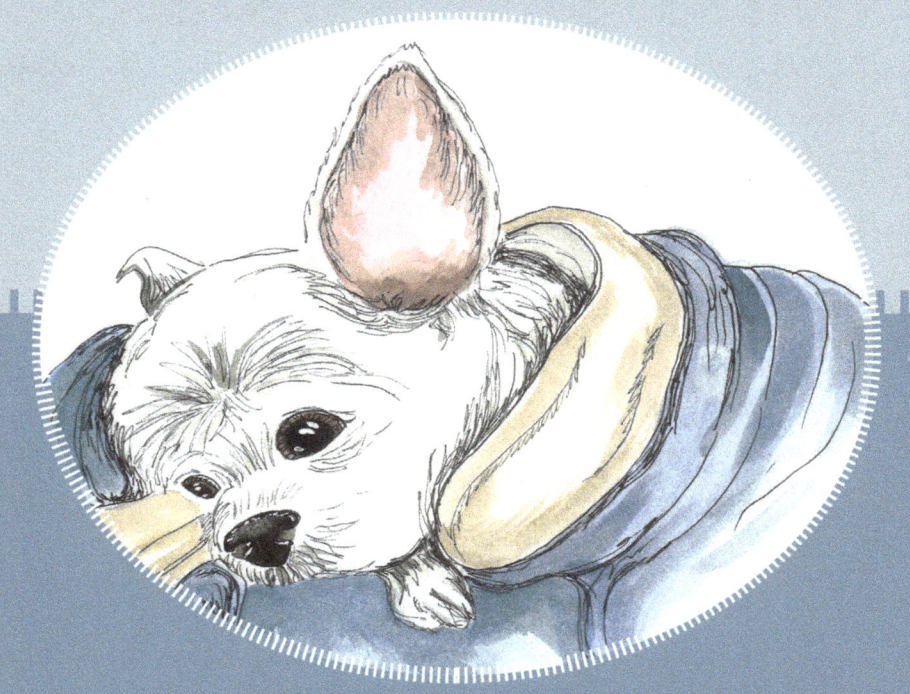

So, Mom took me to the veterinarian. That's a doctor for pups like me and other animals. Have you ever helped take your pets to the vet?

I was afraid to go, but Mom told me that was the only way we were going to find out why I didn't feel well. On the way there, she held me in her lap and sang songs to me.

Once I was there, they did some tests. They were very nice to me and held me and took me for a walk and even gave me a treat!

The next day, the veterinarian told Mom that I had diabetes.

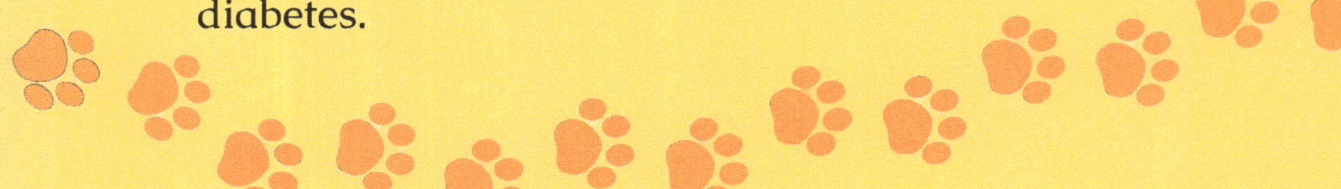

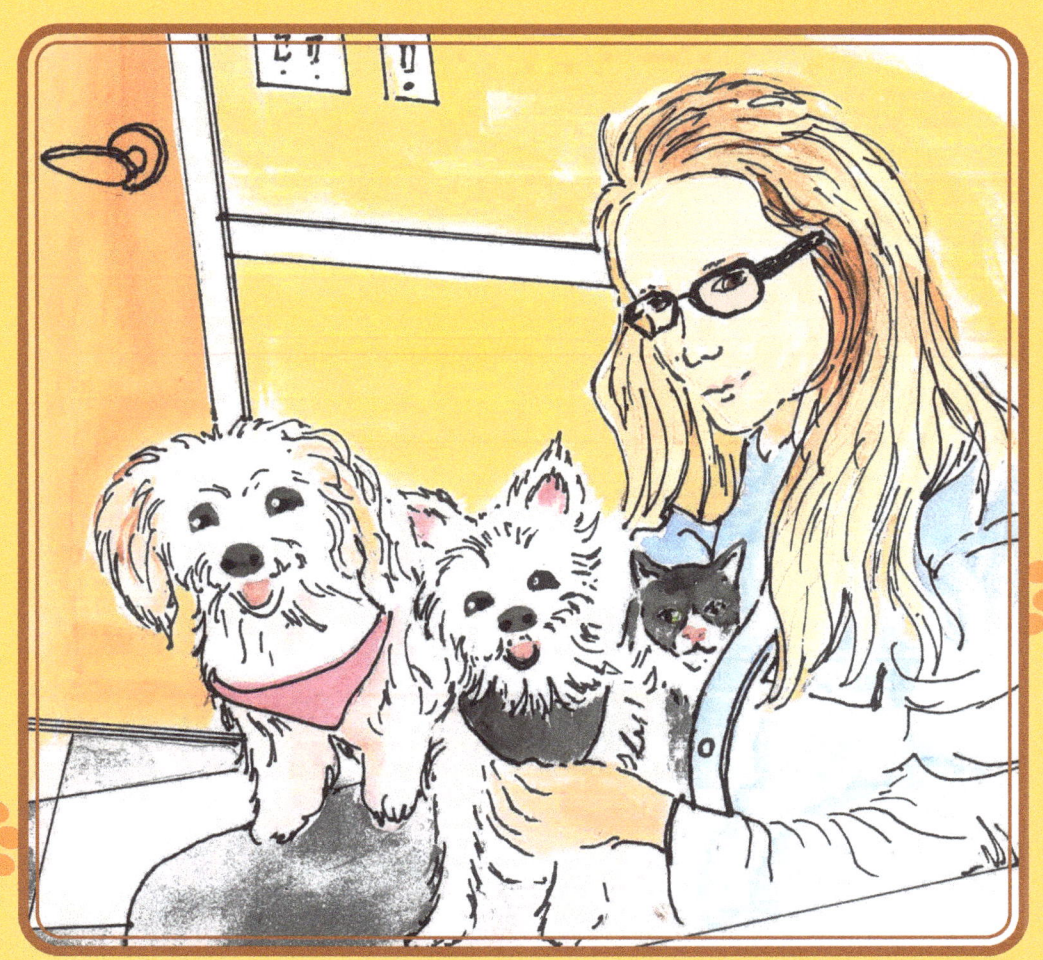

TICA, ME, ZEKE, AND MOM AT THE VET

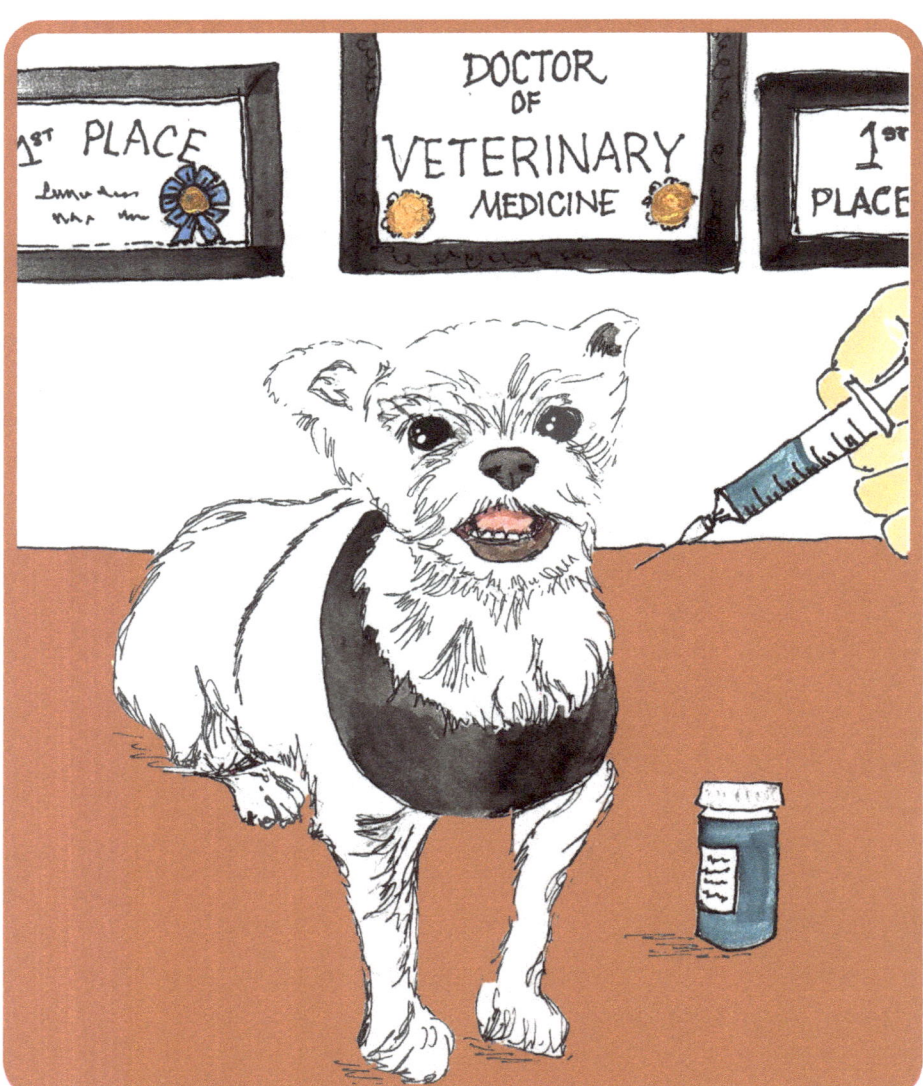

BEING BRAVE !!!!!!!

Diabetes is a condition when there is too much sugar in the blood and not enough insulin. Mom was sad. She didn't like the thought of me not feeling well. The veterinarian told her she didn't do anything wrong; it just was.

He told her that I would need shots of insulin twice a day to help me feel better. Insulin helps keep my blood sugar steady so I feel well and want to play and run and snuggle again.

Mom was nervous about giving me shots because this was new to her and she didn't know how to do it. But the nice lady at the veterinary clinic showed her how to give me my shots. Mom did great and so did I!

When I first started getting the shots, I was very afraid. I growled at mom, which is not like me!! I even tried to bite her a few times!!! I've never done any of that!!! But Mom knew it was just because I was scared.

She kept telling me she was sorry she had to do this, but that it would help me.

She was right! I started to feel better and was less afraid. I have one shot in the morning, after breakfast, and one shot at night after dinner.

Do you have to have shots? Do you take other medicine?

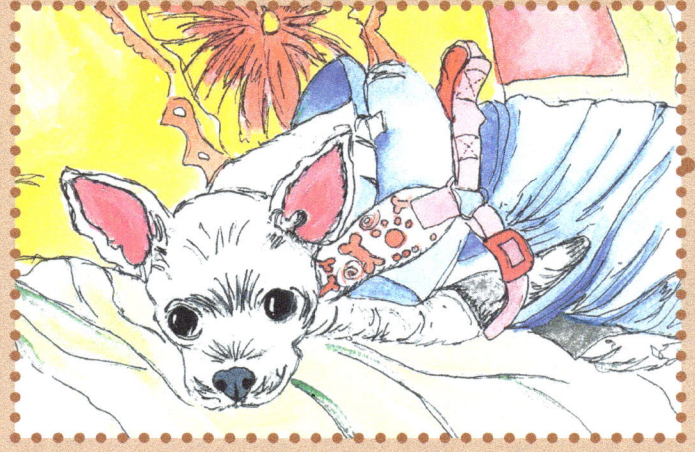

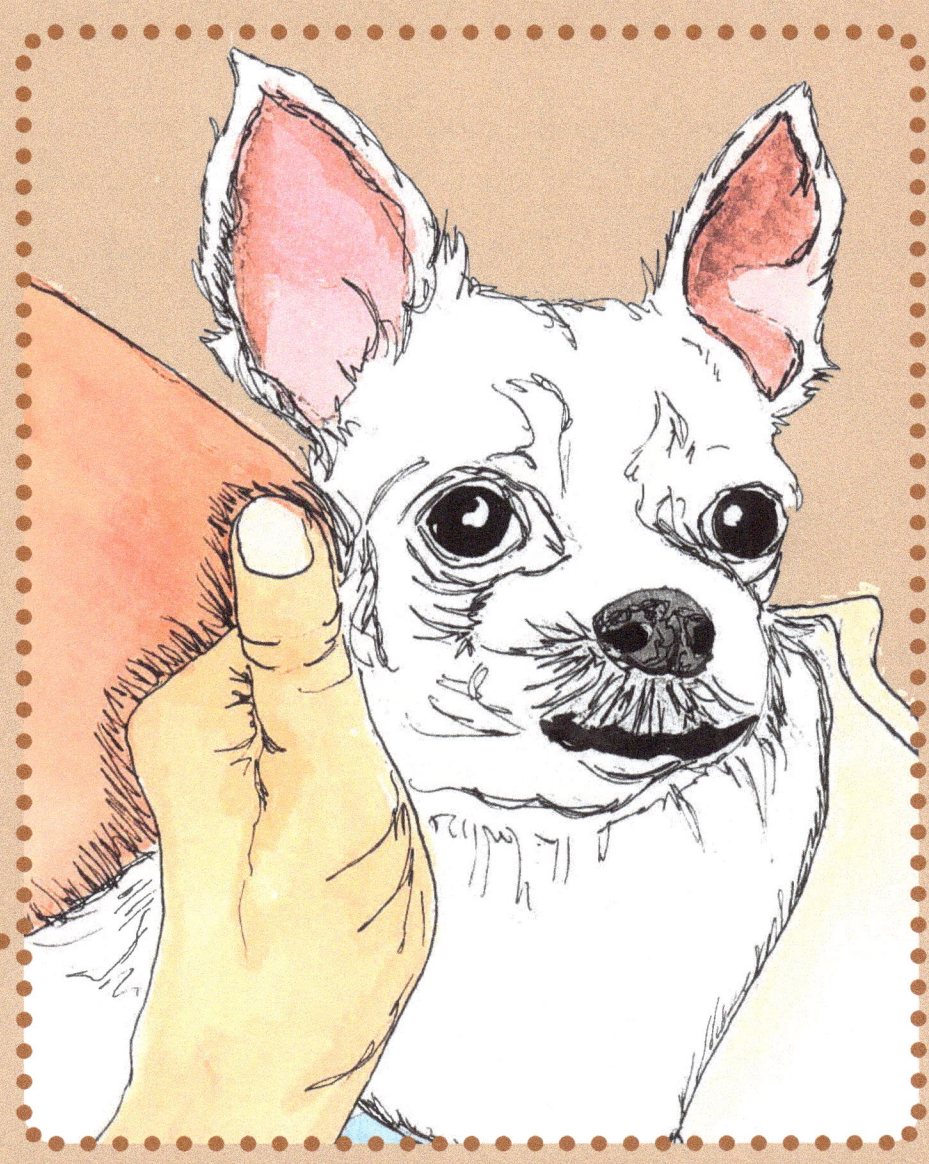

To try to make it a little easier, she gave me some treats to eat while she gave me the shot. She would talk to me, and tell me how brave I am. She sang songs that she made up for me. One of them is

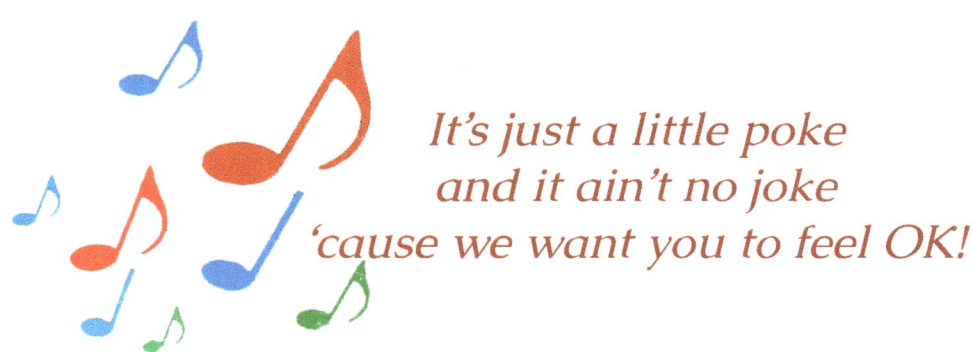

*It's just a little poke
and it ain't no joke
'cause we want you to feel OK!*

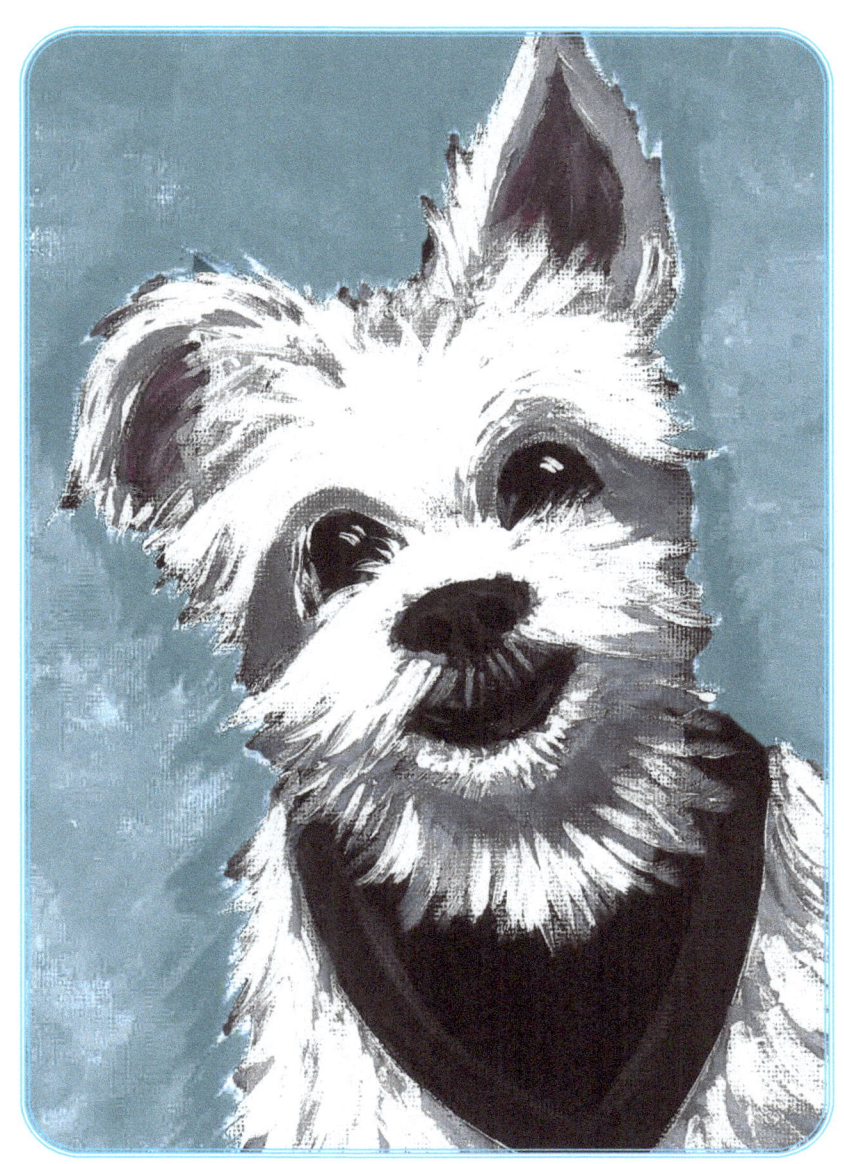

Mom got better at giving me the shots and it went faster and bothered me less. Mom would rub the area where she gave me the shot and tell me she loved me.

It only takes a few seconds and then it is over! When it's all done, Mom says "YAAAAAAAY!!!" and tells me how brave I am. Sometimes I even wag my tail when she gives my shot! That's how far I've come!

And I began to feel a whole lot better!

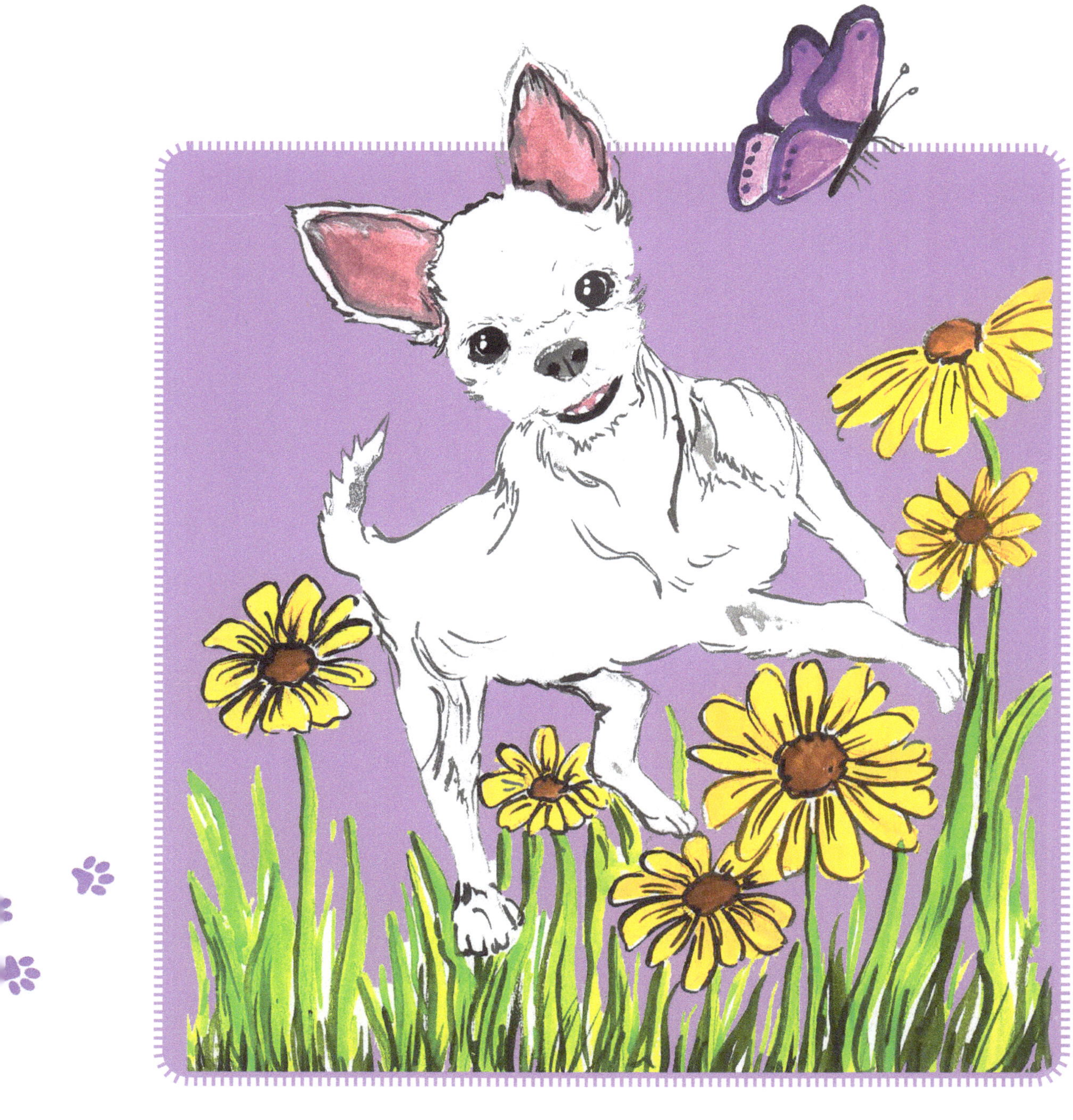

Even after we found out I had diabetes, I still had to go back to the veterinary clinic for checkups, to make sure I was getting the right amount of insulin. I didn't want to go!!! But Mom said it was important, so I went.

Being brave doesn't mean you're not afraid; it means doing the thing you're afraid to do anyway.

Mom said I was a champion and the bravest little pup in the world!

I've also had other medical conditions and even though I'm afraid, I do what the veterinarian and my mom say I need to do, and then I feel better. The veterinarian calls me "scrappy". That means I'm a fighter and I do what I have to do even when I'm afraid.

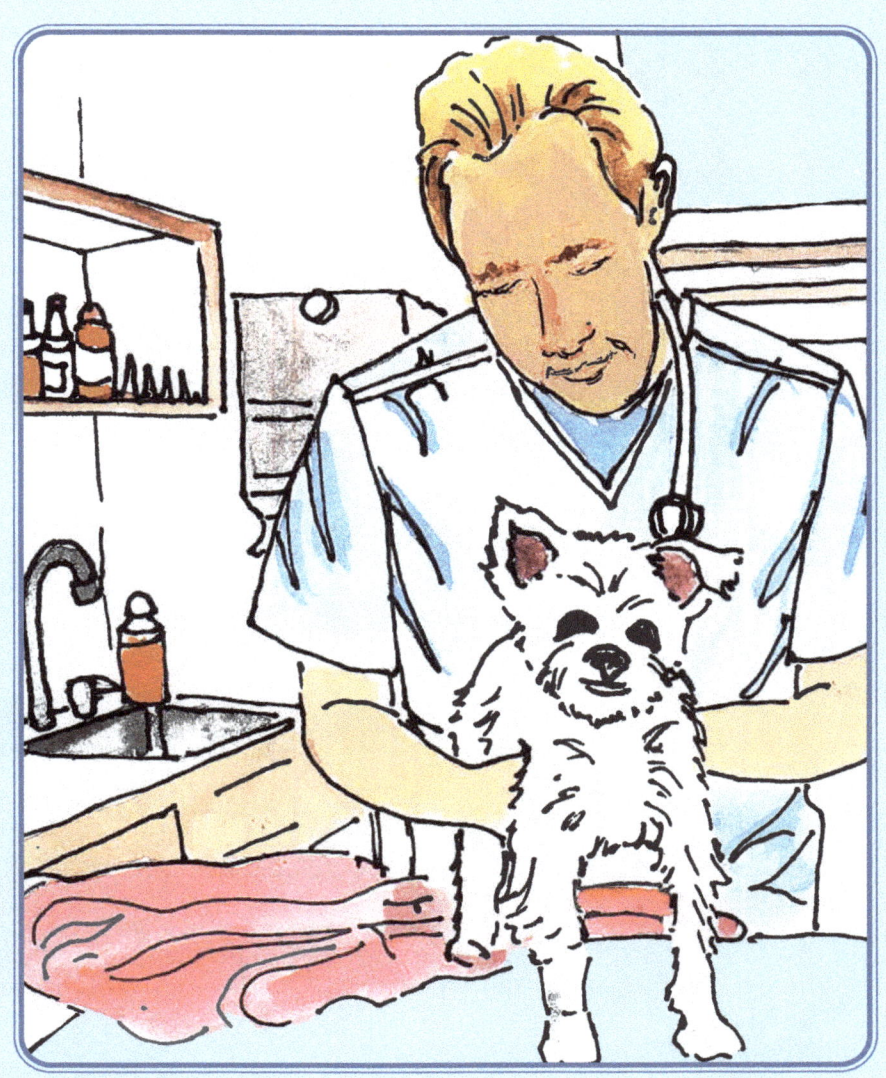

DR. F AND ME

Mom says I've overcome so much and that I'm just as brave as a **firefighter** · · · · · · · · · · · · · · · · · · ·

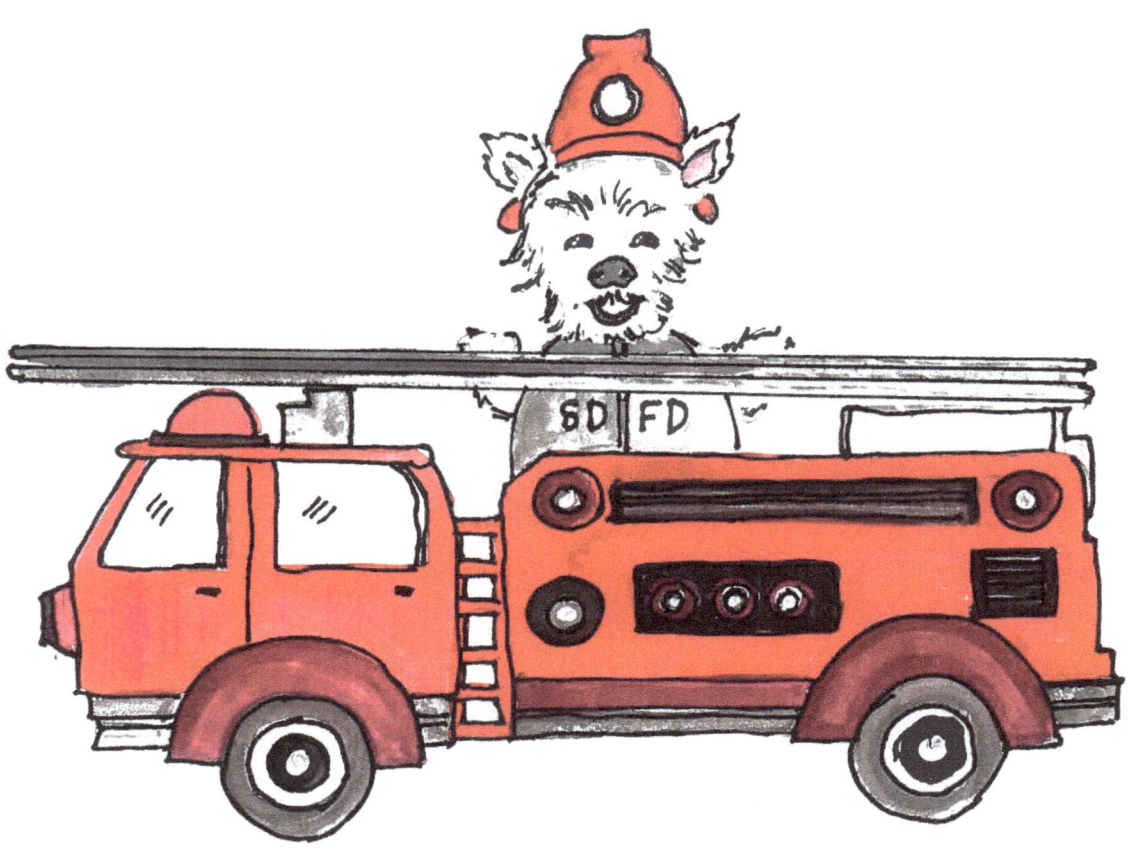

an **astronaut!** ....

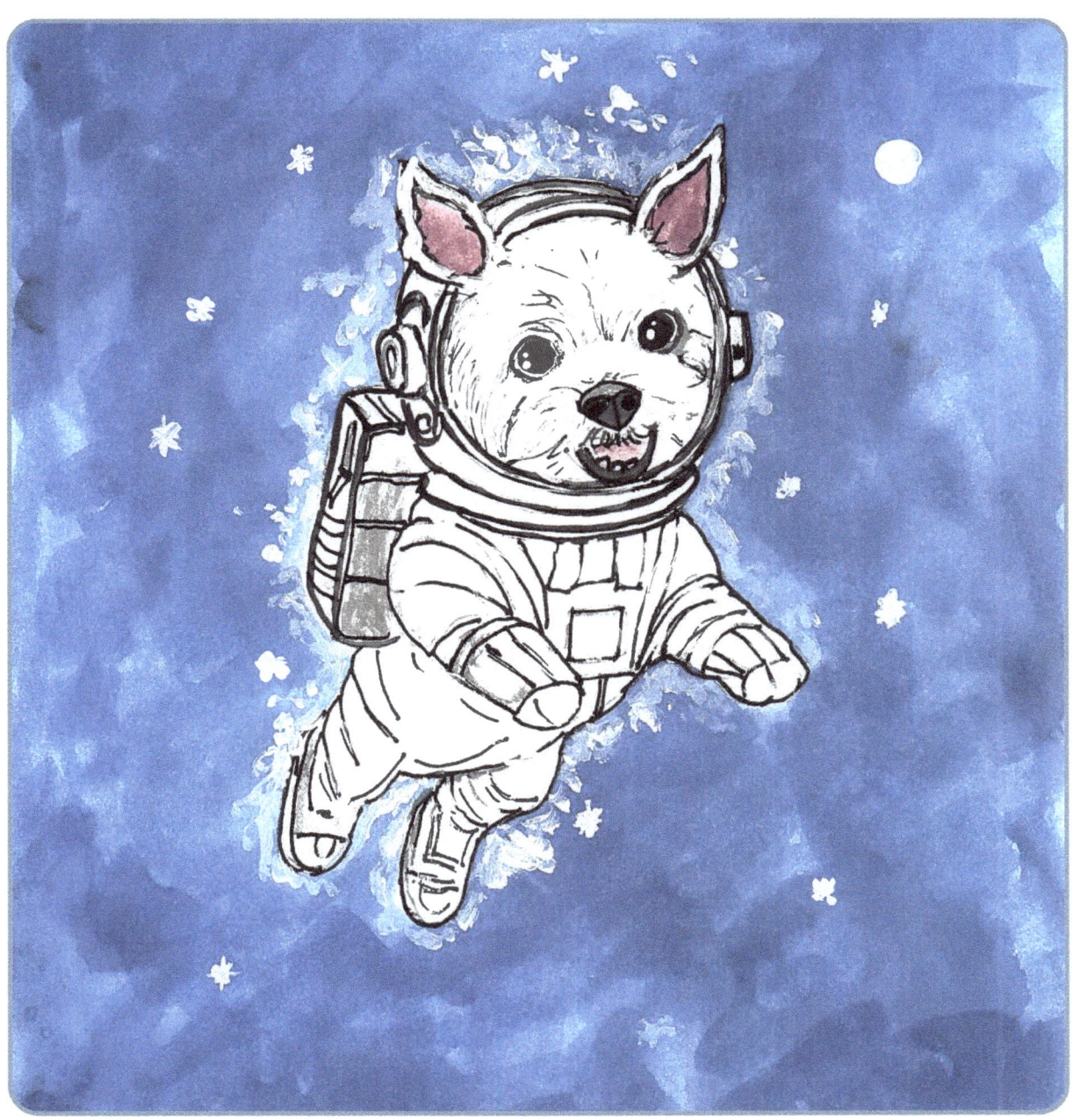

and even a

SUBMARINE CAPTAIN!!!

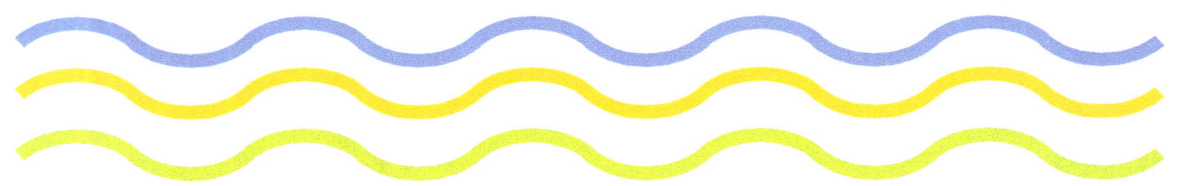

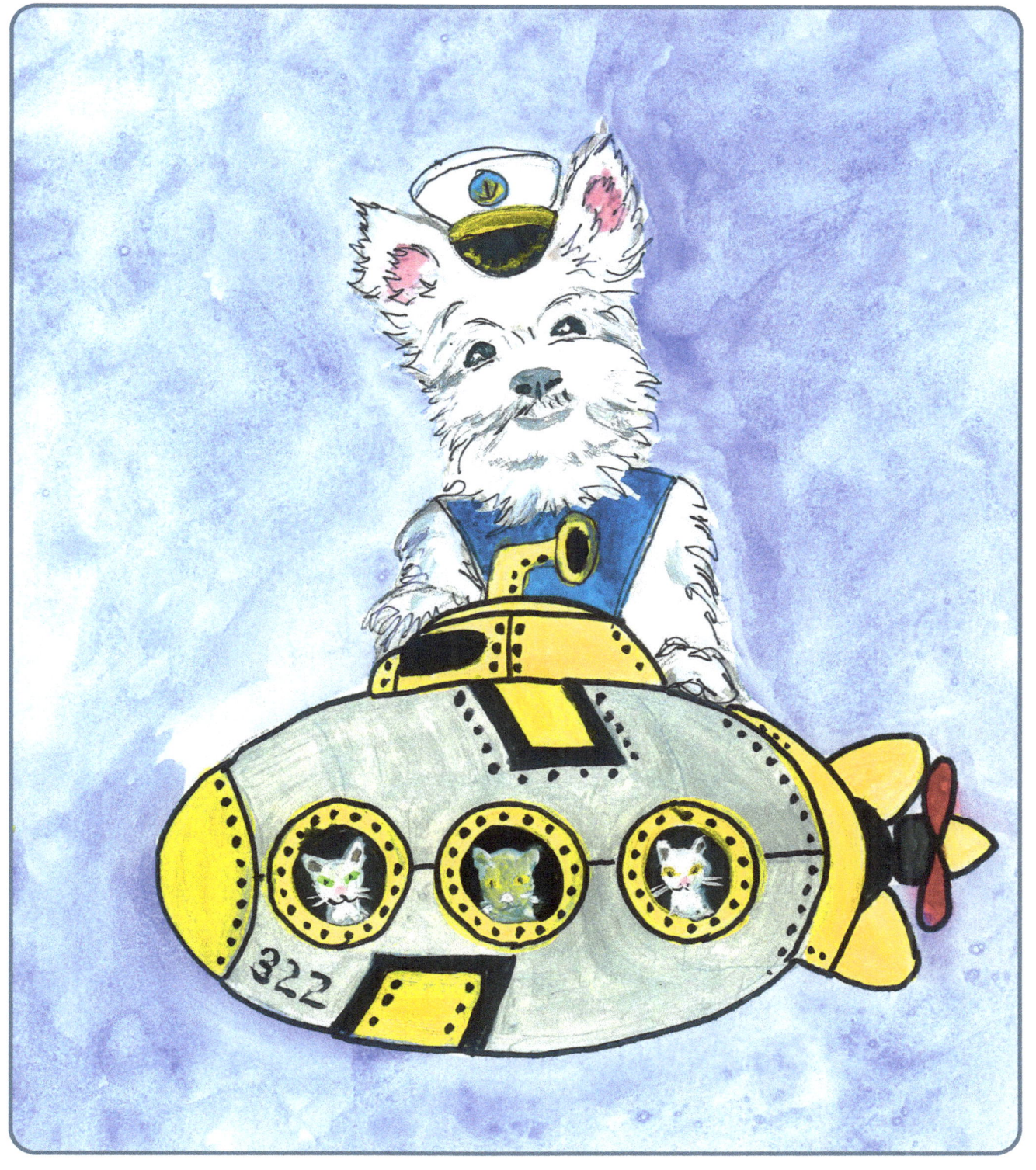

Mom tells me that I have helped her be brave. When she is afraid of doing something, she thinks of me, her little pup who only weighs nine pounds, and everything I have faced, and it gives her the strength to do what she's afraid to do. She says she wants to be brave like Lukas!!!

So, any time you have to do something that you're afraid to do, like get a shot, or take some medicine, or go to the doctor's office, you can say

"I'M BRAVE LIKE LUKAS !!!!"

You can say it really loudly if it helps you!! When you feel like you don't have courage, you can take some from me!! Pretend I am there with you!!

I'll be with you in spirit,
helping you be brave!!

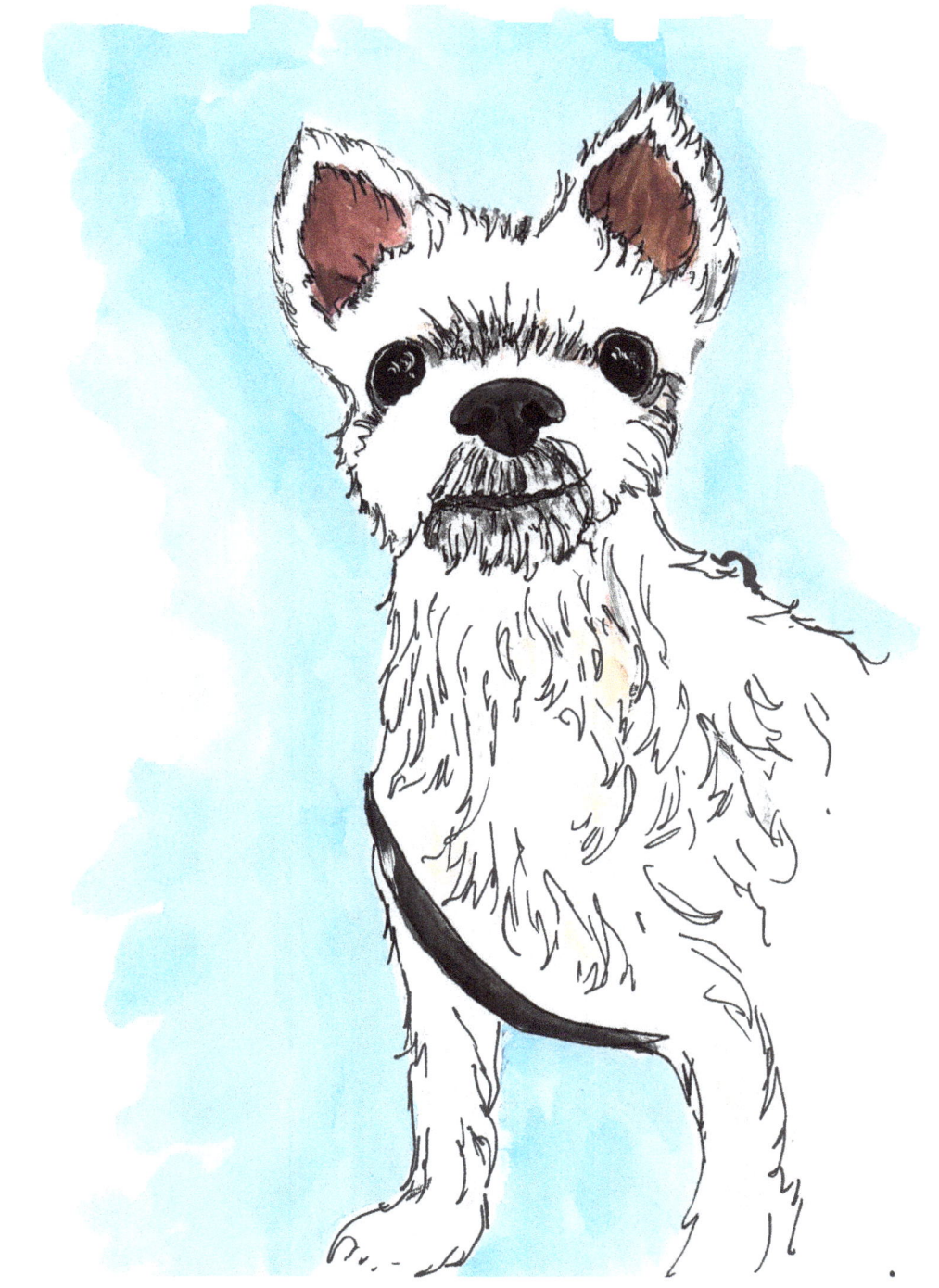

My gang and me . . . .

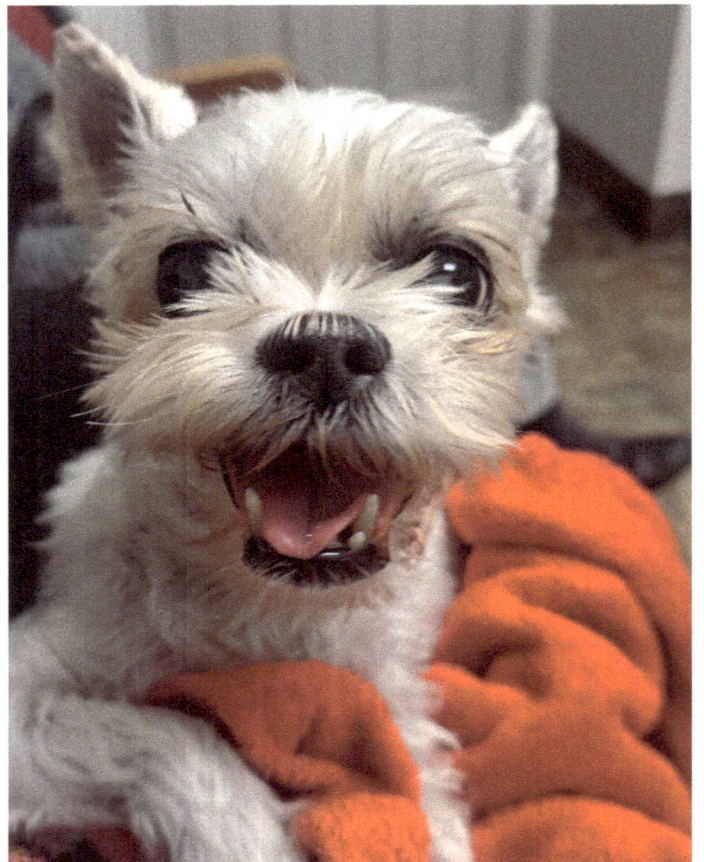
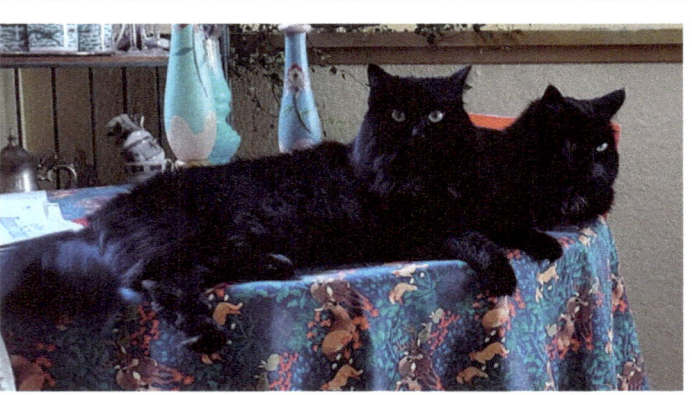
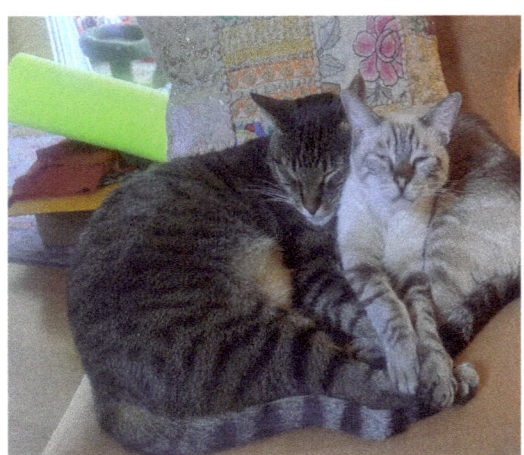
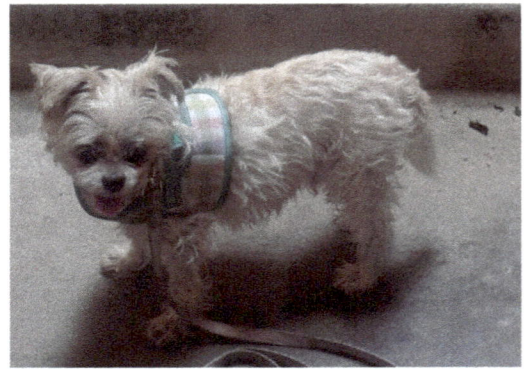
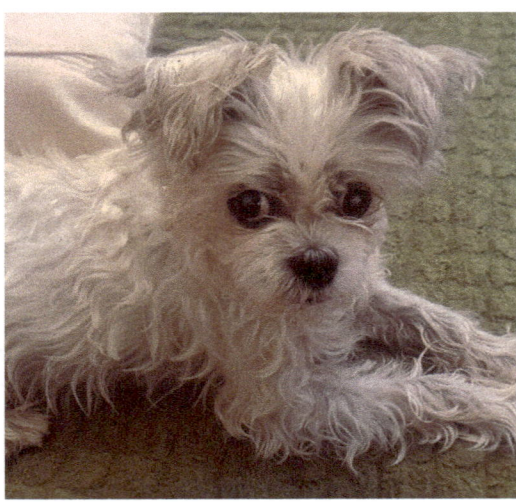

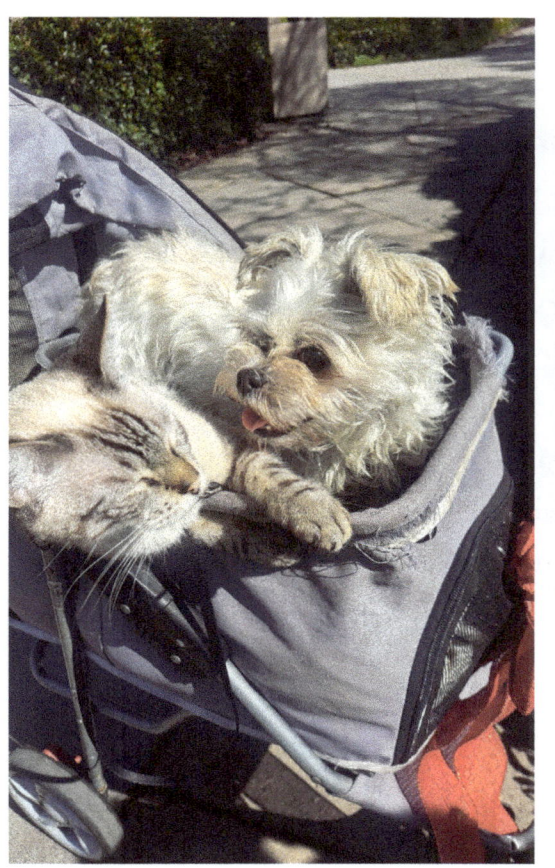
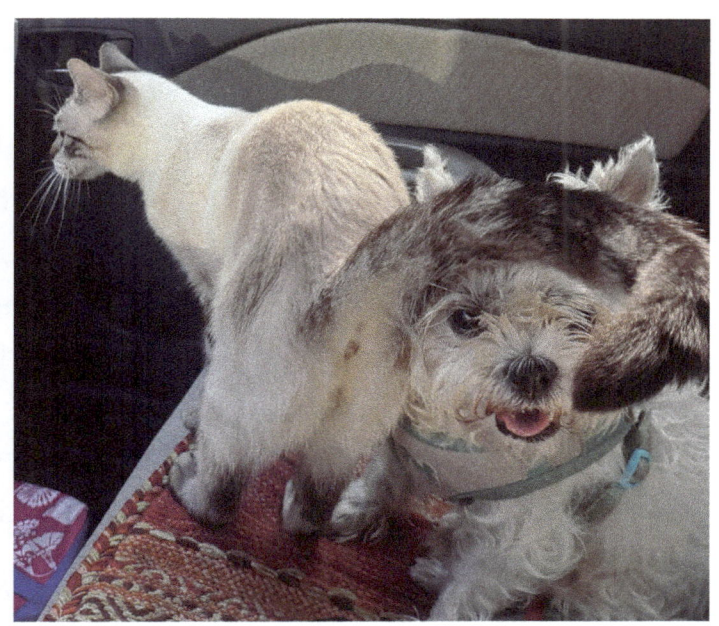
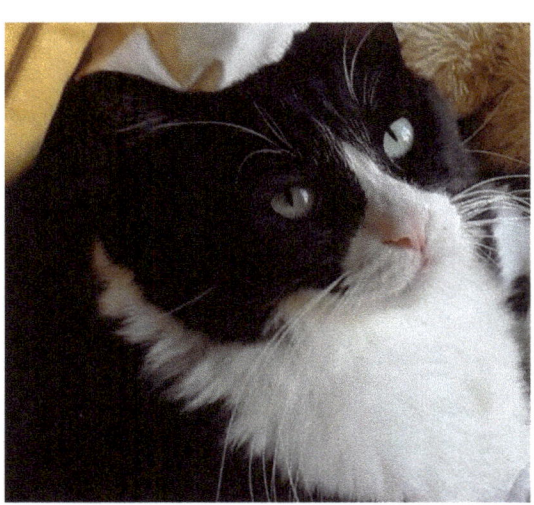
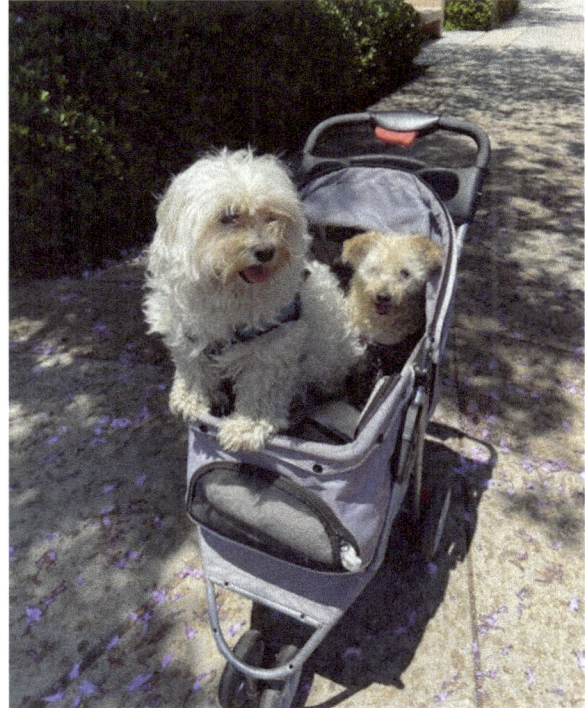

Claudia Krissinger enjoyed teaching Art to high school students during her 35-year teaching career at Susquenita High School. After retirement, wanting to give back, she painted pictures of service dogs for soldiers that were injured in the war because their dogs are such an important part of their lives and recovery. She hopes that children reading this book can take comfort in knowing that Lukas shares their journey with diabetes. She is a proud mother to Dan and grandmother to Alexa and Ava, all joys of her life.

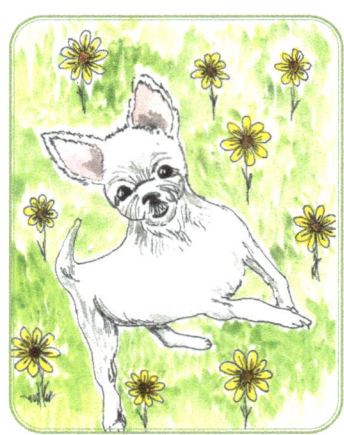

Lukas, his mom Lisa, and the rest of the gang live in their fun little home in San Diego, CA. We love our walks, play time, and treats. Lisa enjoys caring for animals, interior design, the *New York Times* crossword puzzle, military history, and contemplating the next book, possibly about Murray and Jasper solving mysteries!

So stay tuned! And check out the website: www.bravelikelukas.com

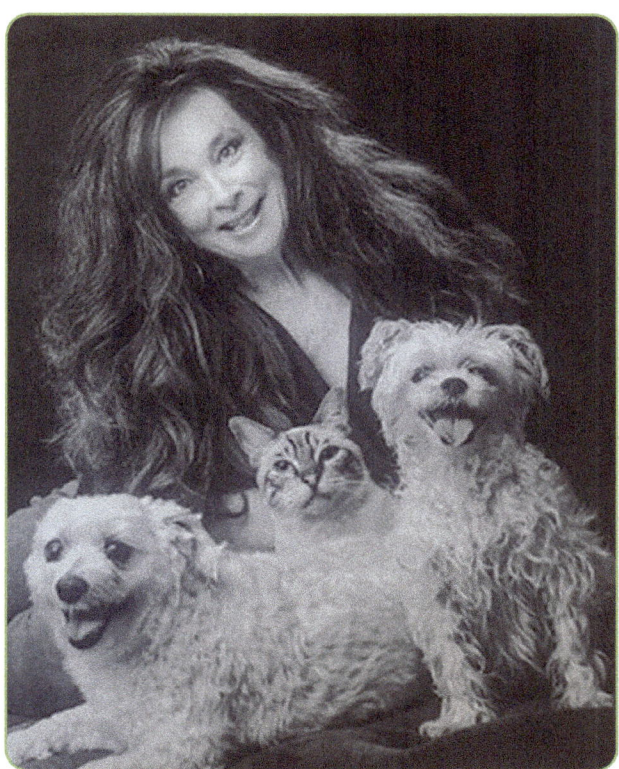

Photo: Debora Cartwright, Del Mar Photographics.

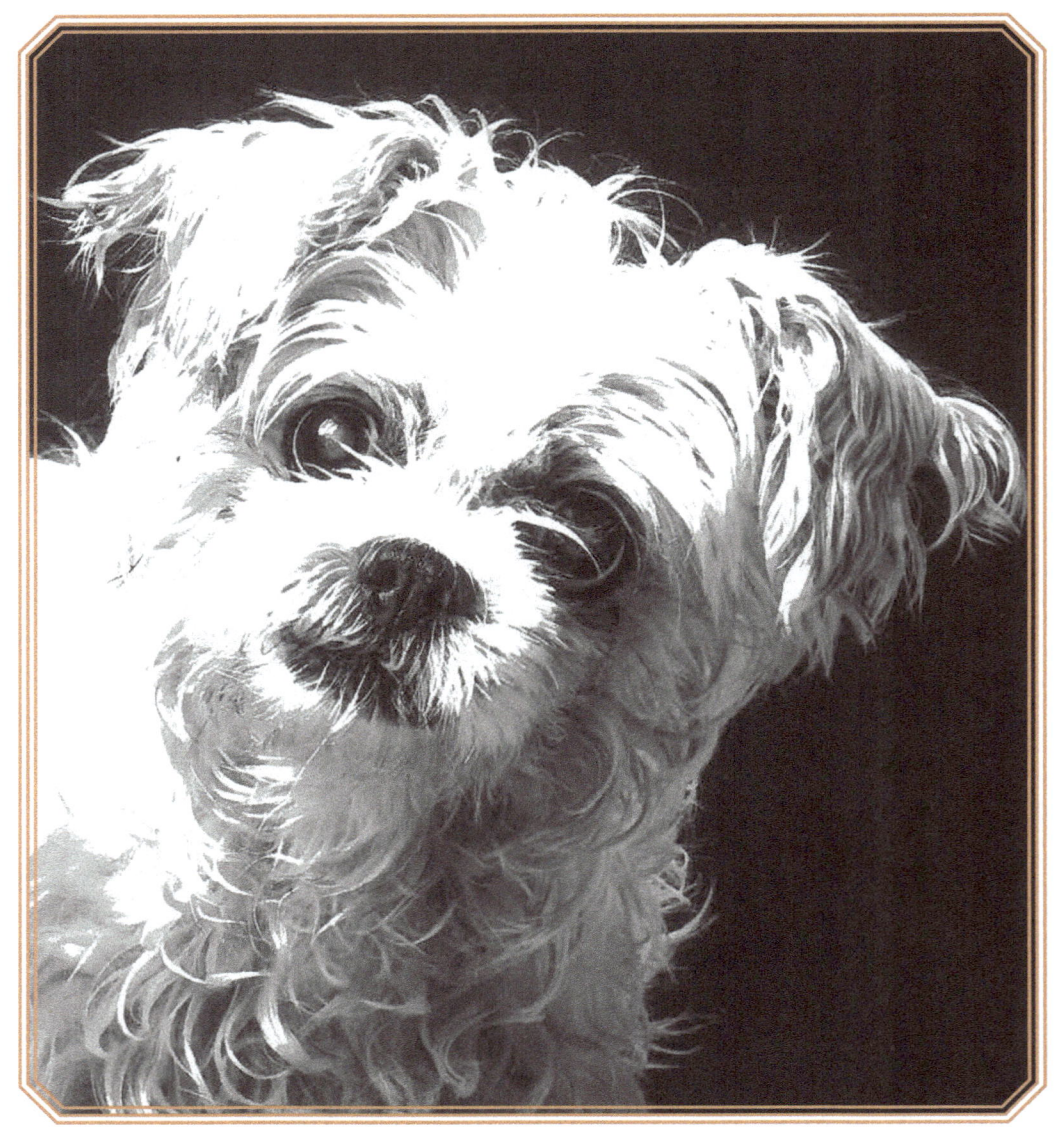

Brave Like Lukas®
www.bravelikelukas.com

I was BRAVE today!

Here is where you can write down all the ways *you* were brave

_____
_____
_____
_____
_____
_____
_____
_____
_____
_____
_____
_____
_____
_____

I was BRAVE today!

Here is where you can write down all the ways *you* were brave

_____
_____
_____
_____
_____
_____
_____
_____
_____
_____
_____
_____
_____
_____
_____
_____
_____
_____

I was BRAVE today!

Here is where you can write down all the ways *you* were brave

www.ingramcontent.com/pod-product-compliance
Lightning Source LLC
Chambersburg PA
CBHW040005040426
42337CB00033B/5231